Table of Contents

Menopause is one point in a continuum of life stages for women and marks the end of their reproductive years. After menopause, a woman cannot become pregnant, except in rare cases when specialized fertility treatments are used.

Most women experience menopause between the ages of 45 and 55 years as a natural part of biological ageing.

Menopause is caused by the loss of ovarian follicular function and a decline in circulating blood oestrogen levels.

The menopausal transition can be gradual, usually beginning with changes in the menstrual cycle. 'Perimenopause' refers to the period from when these signs are first observed and ends one year after the final menstrual period.

Perimenopause can last several years and can affect physical, emotional, mental and social well-being.

A variety of non-hormonal and hormonal interventions can help alleviate perimenopausal symptoms.

Menopause can be a consequence of surgical or medical procedures.

BREAKFAST

1. Quick Taco

Prep Time: 5Minutes

Cook Time: 10Minutes

Servings: 1

Ingredients

- 2 corn tortillas
- 1 tablespoon salsa
- 2 tablespoons shredded reduced-fat Cheddar cheese
- ½ cup liquid egg substitute, such as Egg Beaters

Instructions

1. Top tortillas with salsa and cheese. Heat in the microwave until the cheese is melted, about 30 seconds.

2. Meanwhile coat a small nonstick skillet with cooking spray. Heat over medium heat, add egg substitute and

cook, stirring, until the eggs are cooked through, about 90 seconds. Divide the scrambled egg between the tacos.

Prep Time: 2 Minutes

Cook Time: 8 Minutes

Servings: 1

Ingredients

- 1 cup baby carrots (see Tip)
- ¾ cup fat-free, plain Greek yogurt
- 2 slices reduced-calorie, whole-grain bread, toasted
- ¾ cup low-sodium vegetable juice
- ¾ cup blueberries (Optional)

Instructions

1. Assemble carrots, Greek yogurt, toast on a plate or in separate containers. Serve with low-sodium vegetable juice.
2. Serve with blueberries to complete this balanced meal.

Prep Time: 5 Minutes

Cook Time: 10 Minutes

Servings: 1

Ingredients

- Nonstick cooking spray
- ¼ cup refrigerated or frozen egg product, thawed
- 1/8 to 1/4 teaspoon salt-free southwest chipotle seasoning blend
- 1 whole-wheat flour tortilla
- 2 tablespoons shredded part-skim mozzarella cheese
- 2 tablespoons canned no-salt-added black beans, rinsed and drained
- 2 tablespoons refrigerated fresh pico de gallo or chopped tomato plus more for garnish

Instructions

1. Coat a medium nonstick skillet with nonstick cooking spray. Preheat skillet over medium heat. Add egg to hot skillet; sprinkle with seasoning blend. Cook over

medium heat, without stirring, until egg begins to set on the bottom and around edge. Using a spatula or a large spoon, lift and fold the partially cooked egg so that the uncooked portion flows underneath. Continue cooking over medium heat for 30 to 60 seconds or until egg is cooked through but is still glossy and moist.

2. Immediately spoon cooked egg onto one side of the tortilla. Top with cheese, beans and the 2 tablespoons pico de gallo. Fold tortilla over filling to cover; press gently.

3. Wipe out the same skillet with a paper towel. Coat skillet with cooking spray. Preheat skillet over medium heat. Cook filled tortilla in hot skillet about 2 minutes or until tortilla is browned and filling is heated through, turning once. If desired, top with additional pico de gallo.

Prep Time: 30 Minutes

Cook Time: 30 Minutes

Servings: 6

Ingredients

- 1 cup quick-cooking rolled oats
- ¼ cup unsweetened shredded coconut
- 3 whole pitted Medjool dates
- ¼ cup boiling water
- ⅓ cup cashew butter or peanut butter
- ¼ cup dried apricots, quartered
- 2 tablespoons ground chia seeds or flaxmeal
- 2 tablespoons roasted salted cashews
- ½ teaspoon ground ginger
- ¼ teaspoon salt
- 2 tablespoons finely chopped dark chocolate (Optional)
- 1 (5.3 ounce) container nonfat vanilla Greek yogurt

Instructions

1. Preheat oven to 325 degrees F.

2. Combine oats and coconut in a small shallow baking pan. Bake, stirring once, until the coconut is light brown, 6 to 8 minutes. Cool in the pan on a wire rack.

3. Meanwhile, combine dates and boiling water in a small heatproof bowl. Let stand until softened, about 5 minutes. Drain.

4. Transfer the dates to a food processor and process until chopped. Add the oat mixture, cashew (or peanut) butter, apricots, chia seeds (or flaxmeal), cashews, ginger, and salt. Pulse until the mixture clings together. Stir in chocolate, if using. Shape into 1 1/2-inch balls to make 12 breakfast bites. (See Tips.) Serve with yogurt for dipping.

Prep Time: 10 Minutes

Cook Time: 10 Minutes

Servings: 1

Ingredients

- 1 tablespoon roasted garlic avocado-oil mayonnaise
- 1 everything bagel thin, toasted
- 1 slice Monterey Jack cheese
- ¼ avocado, sliced
- 2 tablespoons alfalfa sprouts
- 1 large egg, fried
- 2 tablespoons thinly sliced red onion

Instructions

1. Spread mayonnaise on 1 bagel thin half. Top with cheese, avocado, sprouts, fried egg and onion. Top with the remaining bagel thin half.

Prep Time: 30 Minutes

Cook Time: 1hr 50 Minutes

Servings: 20

Ingredients

- 6 cups old-fashioned rolled oats
- 1 cup chopped almonds
- 1 cup chopped walnuts
- 1 cup raw, unsalted pepitas
- ½ cup maple syrup
- 6 tablespoons canola oil
- ¼ cup honey
- 1 teaspoon ground cinnamon
- 1 teaspoon vanilla extract
- ½ teaspoon salt

Instructions

1. Preheat oven to 325 degrees F. Line a roasting pan or large baking sheet with parchment paper.

2. Combine oats, almonds, walnuts and pepitas in a large bowl. Whisk maple syrup, oil, honey, cinnamon, vanilla and salt in a medium bowl until blended. Pour over the oat mixture and toss to coat. Spread the mixture in the prepared pan.

3. Bake, stirring every 15 minutes, until lightly and evenly browned and starting to dry out, 50 minutes to 1 hour. Let cool completely in the pan before serving or storing.

Prep Time: 30 Minutes

Cook Time: 1hr 50 Minutes

Servings: 20

Ingredients

- 4 crisp apples, such as Jazz or Pink Lady, divided
- 1 cup steel-cut oats
- 4 cups water
- 3 tablespoons packed brown sugar, divided
- ½ teaspoon ground cinnamon
- ¼ teaspoon salt
- ½ cup nonfat plain Greek yogurt

Instructions

1. Shred 2 apples using the large holes of a box grater, leaving the core behind.
2. Heat a large saucepan over medium-high heat. Add oats and cook, stirring, until lightly toasted, about 2 minutes. Add water and the shredded apples; bring to

a boil. Reduce heat to maintain a simmer and cook, stirring frequently, for 10 minutes.

3. Meanwhile, chop the remaining 2 apples.
4. After the oats have cooked for 10 minutes, stir in the chopped apples, 2 tablespoons brown sugar, cinnamon and salt; continue cooking, stirring occasionally, until the apples are tender and the oatmeal is quite thick, 15 to 20 minutes more. Divide the oatmeal among 4 bowls. Top each portion with 2 tablespoons yogurt and 3/4 teaspoon brown sugar.

Prep Time: 30Minutes

Cook Time: 1hr 50Minutes

Servings: 2

Ingredients

- 1 cup unsweetened soy milk
- 1 cup frozen strawberries
- 1 cup chopped kale
- 1 tablespoon natural peanut butter
- 1 tablespoon honey
- 1 teaspoon vanilla extract
- 2-4 ice cubes

Instructions

1. Combine soymilk, strawberries, kale, peanut butter, honey, vanilla and ice cubes in a blender. Puree until smooth.

Prep Time: 25 Minutes

Cook Time: 25 Minutes

Servings: 4

Ingredients

- 4 slices bacon, chopped
- 1 cup chopped fresh mushrooms
- ½ cup chopped green sweet pepper (1 small)
- ¼ teaspoon chili powder
- ¼ teaspoon ground black pepper
- ⅛ teaspoon salt
- 1 cup refrigerated or frozen egg product, thawed
- ¼ cup chopped seeded tomato
- Few drops bottled hot pepper sauce
- 4 (8 inch) flour tortillas, warmed

Instructions

1. In a large nonstick skillet, cook bacon over medium heat until crisp. Using a slotted spoon, remove bacon from skillet, reserving 1 tablespoon of the drippings in

the skillet (discard the remaining drippings). Drain bacon on paper towels.

2. Add mushrooms, sweet pepper, chili powder, pepper, and salt to the reserved drippings in skillet; cook and stir about 3 minutes or until vegetables are tender.

3. Pour egg over vegetable mixture in skillet. Using a spatula or a large spoon, lift and fold egg mixture so that the uncooked portion flows underneath. Continue cooking over medium heat about 2 minutes or until egg is cooked through but is still glossy and moist. Stir in cooked bacon, tomato, and hot pepper sauce. Divide egg mixture among tortillas; roll up tortillas.

Prep Time: 25Minutes

Cook Time: 45Minutes

Servings: 6

Ingredients:

- 3 small-to-medium russet potatoes (6-8 ounces each)
- 2 tablespoons butter
- ½ cup finely chopped red bell pepper
- ¼ cup sliced scallions
- 3 large eggs, beaten
- ¼ teaspoon salt
- ¼ teaspoon ground pepper
- ½ cup shredded Mexican cheese blend

Instructions

1. Prick potatoes with a fork in several places. Microwave on High for 5 minutes. Turnover and continue cooking on High until tender all the way through, about 4 minutes more. (Alternatively, bake at 350 degrees F until tender, 50 minutes to 1 hour.) When cool enough

to handle, cut the potatoes in half lengthwise and scoop out the flesh, leaving a 1/4-inch border. Chop enough of the potato flesh to equal about 1 cup. (Save the remaining potato for another use or discard.)

2. Heat butter in a large nonstick skillet over medium-high heat. Add bell pepper, scallions and the chopped potato. Cook, stirring often, until the pepper softens, 3 to 4 minutes. Add eggs, salt and pepper and cook, stirring, until set, 1 to 2 minutes. Remove from heat. Fold in cheese.

3. Generously stuff each potato half with about 1/2 cup of the egg mixture. Let cool completely, then individually wrap with heavy-duty foil. Refrigerate or store in a cold cooler for up to 1 day.

4. Prepare a campfire and let it burn down to the coals. Place the wrapped potato boats 4 to 6 inches above the coals; cook, turning once or twice, until steaming hot and completely heated through, 10 to 15 minutes. Open carefully. (Alternatively, unwrap and reheat in the microwave.)

Prep Time: 20 Minutes

Cook Time: 1hr 10 Minutes

Servings: 10

Ingredients

- 3 teaspoons extra-virgin olive oil, divided
- 12 ounces bulk turkey sausage
- 1 ½ cups chopped yellow onion
- 1 cup chopped red bell pepper
- 2 cloves garlic, finely chopped
- 8 large eggs
- 1 ½ cups whole milk
- 2 teaspoons chili powder
- ½ teaspoon cayenne pepper
- ¼ teaspoon ground pepper
- 1 (28 ounce) package frozen potato tots
- ¾ cup shredded sharp Cheddar cheese
- 1 tablespoon chopped fresh chives

Instructions

1. Preheat oven to 350°F. Lightly coat a 9-by-13-inch baking dish with cooking spray. Heat 2 teaspoons oil in a large nonstick skillet over medium-high heat. Add sausage; cook, stirring and breaking up the meat with a wooden spoon, until browned, 5 to 6 minutes. Transfer to a paper-towel-lined plate. Do not wipe the skillet clean.

2. Add the remaining 1 teaspoon oil to the skillet; heat over medium-high heat. Add onion and bell pepper; cook, stirring occasionally, until tender, about 7 minutes. Add garlic; cook, stirring often, until fragrant, about 1 minute. Add the vegetables to the reserved sausage.

3. Whisk eggs, milk, chili powder, cayenne and pepper in a large bowl. Add the sausage-vegetable mixture; stir until combined. Pour into the prepared baking dish. Top evenly with potato tots, arranging them in a single layer. Sprinkle with cheese.

4. Bake until the casserole is set and the cheese is golden brown, 40 to 45 minutes. Let stand for 10 minutes. Sprinkle with chives before serving.

Prep Time: 35 Minutes

Cook Time: 1hr 35 Minutes

Servings: 6

Ingredients

- 2 dried ancho chiles (about 1 ounce)
- 2 ½ cups boiling water
- 8 ounces scallions, trimmed, plus more for garnish
- 2 tablespoons lime juice
- ½ teaspoon salt, divided
- ½ teaspoon ground pepper, divided
- 6 large eggs
- 3 slices thick-cut bacon, chopped
- ¾ cup shredded cheese, such as Monterey Jack
- 6 corn or flour tortillas, warmed
- Shredded red cabbage & lime wedges for serving

Instructions

1. Place chiles in a heatproof bowl and cover with boiling water. Cover and let stand until softened, about 1 hour.

2. Separate scallion whites and greens and cut into 4-inch pieces. Heat a large cast-iron skillet over high heat. Cook the whites, turning occasionally, until almost entirely blackened, about 5 minutes. Transfer to a plate. Cook the greens until lightly charred, 1 to 2 minutes. Transfer to the plate and let cool.

3. Drain the chiles, reserving the water. Remove and discard the stems and seeds. Transfer the chiles to a food processor and add 1/4 cup of the reserved water, the scallions, lime juice and 1/4 teaspoon each salt and pepper. Puree until smooth.

4. Whisk eggs with the remaining 1/4 teaspoon each salt and pepper in a medium bowl.

5. Wipe out the pan to remove any blackened bits. Add bacon and cook over medium heat, stirring occasionally, until just starting to brown, 2 to 5 minutes. Add the eggs and cook, stirring, until just set, 1 to 3 minutes. Remove from heat. Sprinkle the eggs with cheese and cover until it melts, 1 to 3 minutes.

6. Divide the eggs among tortillas. Serve topped with the salsa and more scallions, cabbage and lime wedges, if desired.

Prep Time: 20 Minutes

Cook Time: 2hr 15 Minutes

Servings: 6

Ingredients

- 1 (16 ounce) package frozen shredded hash browns, thawed
- 1 ¼ cups finely shredded Cheddar-Jack cheese, divided
- 6 large eggs
- ½ cup whole milk
- 1 teaspoon garlic powder
- ¼ teaspoon salt
- ¼ teaspoon ground pepper
- 4 center-cut bacon slices, cooked and crumbled

Instructions

1. Place thawed hash browns in a clean kitchen towel. Squeeze until most of the moisture has been released. Place the hash browns in a medium bowl; add 1/2 cup

cheese and toss to combine. Lightly coat a 9-inch pie pan with cooking spray. Press the hash brown mixture into the bottom and up the sides of the pan, making sure there are no holes. Freeze until firm, about 1 hour.

2. Preheat oven to 425°F. Remove the pie pan from the freezer and let stand at room temperature while the oven preheats. Bake until the crust is starting to turn golden brown around the edges, about 20 minutes. Let cool slightly on a wire rack, about 10 minutes. Reduce oven temperature to 375°F.

3. Meanwhile, whisk eggs, milk, garlic powder, salt and pepper together in a medium bowl until well blended. Stir in bacon and the remaining 3/4 cup cheese. Pour the mixture into the warm crust. Bake until the egg mixture is set and the top is light golden brown, 25 to 30 minutes. Let the quiche cool for 5 minutes before slicing and serving.

Prep Time: 15 Minutes

Cook Time: 1hr 5 Minutes

Servings: 16

Ingredients

- 4 cups sweetened oat cereal flakes with raisins
- ¾ cup quick-cooking rolled oats
- ½ cup all-purpose flour
- ½ cup snipped dried apples
- 2 eggs, slightly beaten
- ⅓ cup honey
- ⅓ cup chunky peanut butter
- ¼ cup butter, melted, or cooking oil

Instructions

1. Preheat oven to 325 degrees F. Line a 9x9-inch baking pan with foil. Coat the foil with nonstick cooking spray; set aside.
2. Combine cereal, rolled oats, flour, and dried apples in a large bowl. Set aside.

3. Stir together eggs, honey, peanut butter, and melted butter in a small bowl. Pour over the cereal mixture. Mix well. Transfer the mixture to the prepared pan. Using the back of a large spoon, press the mixture firmly into the pan.

4. Bake in preheated oven for 28 to 30 minutes or until the edges are browned. Cool completely on a wire rack. Cut into bars using a serrated knife.

Prep Time: 15 Minutes

Cook Time: 25 Minutes

Servings: 4

Ingredients:

- 3 slices center-cut bacon
- 1 tablespoon extra-virgin olive oil, plus more if needed
- 3 large cloves garlic, minced
- 1 pound spinach (about 16 cups), tough stems removed
- 1 teaspoon red-wine vinegar
- ½ teaspoon ground pepper, divided
- ¼ teaspoon salt
- 4 large slices country-style whole-wheat bread (3/4-1 inch thick)
- 4 large eggs

Instructions

1. Preheat oven to 425 degrees F. Coat a large baking sheet with cooking spray.

2. Cook bacon in a large cast-iron skillet over medium heat until crisp, 7 to 9 minutes. Drain on paper towels. Pour the bacon fat into a small heatproof bowl. If necessary, add oil to make 2 tablespoons.

3. Meanwhile, heat 1 tablespoon oil in a large saucepan over medium heat. Add garlic and cook, stirring, about 30 seconds. Add spinach by the handful and cook, stirring, until wilted, about 5 minutes. Transfer to a colander; press out excess liquid. Return the spinach to the pan and season with vinegar, 1/4 teaspoon pepper and salt.

4. Cut a 3 1/2-inch hole in the middle of each slice of bread. (Save the rounds for another use, if desired.) Heat 1 tablespoon of the reserved bacon fat in the skillet over medium-high heat. Cook 2 slices of bread, pressing with a spatula, until lightly browned, 1 to 3 minutes per side. Transfer to the prepared baking sheet. Repeat with the remaining fat and bread. Fill each hole with spinach. Make a deep well in the spinach and break an egg into each well.

5. Bake, rotating the baking sheet 180 degrees about halfway through, 10 to 14 minutes for soft-set yolks. Serve sprinkled with crumbled bacon and the remaining 1/4 teaspoon pepper.

Prep Time: 40 Minutes

Cook Time: 40 Minutes

Servings: 1

Ingredients

- ¾ cup white whole-wheat flour
- 1 ½ teaspoons baking soda
- ¼ teaspoon salt plus a pinch, divided
- 1 ½ cups reduced-fat milk
- 2 large eggs, divided
- 1 ½ tablespoons extra-virgin olive oil
- ⅛ teaspoon ground pepper
- 2 teaspoons minced fresh chives (Optional)
- 1 slice bacon, cooked
- 1 teaspoon pure maple syrup

Instructions

1. Whisk flour, baking soda and 1/4 teaspoon salt in a medium bowl. Whisk milk, 1 egg and oil in a small

bowl. Add the milk mixture to the dry ingredients and whisk until smooth.

2. Coat a medium nonstick skillet with cooking spray; heat over medium heat. Ladle 1/3 cup batter into the center of the pan. Immediately tilt and rotate the pan to spread the batter evenly over the bottom. Cook until the underside is golden brown, 1 1/2 to 2 minutes. Using a heatproof silicone or rubber spatula, lift the edge, then quickly grab the pancake with your fingers and flip it over. Cook until the second side is golden brown, about 1 minute more. Slide onto a plate. Repeat with the remaining batter, spraying the pan as needed and stacking pancakes as you go, to make 8 pancakes total.

3. Wipe out the skillet and lightly coat it with cooking spray; heat over medium heat. Whisk the remaining egg, the remaining pinch of salt, pepper and chives (if using) in a small bowl. Pour into the pan and cook, gently stirring, until set, 2 to 3 minutes.

4. To assemble a wrap, layer the egg across the bottom third of 1 warm pancake. Top with bacon, drizzle with syrup and roll up. Save the remaining pancakes for another time.

Prep Time: 5 Minutes

Cook Time: 20 Minutes

Servings: 4

Ingredients

- 4 cups frozen shredded hash brown potatoes
- 2 cups finely chopped baby spinach
- ½ cup finely chopped onion
- 1 tablespoon minced fresh ginger
- 1 tablespoon curry powder
- ½ teaspoon salt
- ¼ cup extra-virgin olive oil
- 1 15-ounce can chickpeas, rinsed
- 1 cup chopped zucchini
- 4 large eggs

Instructions

1. Combine potatoes, spinach, onion, ginger, curry powder and salt in a large bowl.

2. Heat oil in a large nonstick skillet over medium-high heat. Add the potato mixture and press into a layer. Cook, without stirring, until crispy and golden brown on the bottom, 3 to 5 minutes.

3. Reduce heat to medium-low. Fold in chickpeas and zucchini, breaking up chunks of potato, until just combined. Press back into an even layer. Carve out 4 "wells" in the mixture. Break eggs, one at a time, into a cup and slip one into each indentation. Cover and continue cooking until the eggs are set, 4 to 5 minutes for soft-set yolks.

Prep Time: 10 Minutes

Cook Time: 50 Minutes

Servings: 6

Ingredients

- 2 tablespoons fine dry breadcrumbs
- 1 pound thin asparagus
- 1 ½ teaspoons extra-virgin olive oil
- 2 onions, chopped
- 1 red bell pepper, chopped
- 2 cloves garlic, minced
- ½ teaspoon salt, divided
- ½ cup water
- Freshly ground pepper, to taste
- 4 large eggs
- 2 large egg whites
- 1 cup part-skim ricotta cheese
- 1 tablespoon chopped fresh parsley
- ½ cup shredded Gruyère cheese

Instructions

1. Preheat oven to 325 degrees F. Coat a 10-inch pie pan or ceramic quiche dish with cooking spray. Sprinkle with breadcrumbs, tapping out the excess.

2. Snap tough ends off asparagus. Slice off the top 2 inches of the tips and reserve. Cut the stalks into 1/2-inch-long slices.

3. Heat oil in a large nonstick skillet over medium-high heat. Add onions, bell pepper, garlic and 1/4 teaspoon salt; cook, stirring, until softened, 5 to 7 minutes.

4. Add water and the asparagus stalks to the skillet. Cook, stirring, until the asparagus is tender and the liquid has evaporated, about 7 minutes (the mixture should be very dry). Season with salt and pepper. Arrange the vegetables in an even layer in the prepared pan.

5. Whisk eggs and egg whites in a large bowl. Add ricotta, parsley, the remaining 1/4 teaspoon salt and pepper; whisk to blend. Pour the egg mixture over the vegetables, gently shaking the pan to distribute. Scatter the reserved asparagus tips over the top and sprinkle with Gruyere.

6. Bake the frittata until a knife inserted in the center comes out clean, about 35 minutes. Let stand for 5 minutes before serving.

Prep Time: 5 Minutes

Cook Time: 15 Minutes

Servings: 4

Ingredients

- 2 tablespoons extra-virgin olive oil
- 1 ½ cups thinly sliced red onion
- 1 ½ cups chopped zucchini
- 7 large eggs, beaten
- ½ teaspoon salt
- ¼ teaspoon freshly ground pepper
- ⅔ cup pearl-size or baby fresh mozzarella balls (about 4 ounces)
- 3 tablespoons chopped soft sun-dried tomatoes
- ¼ cup thinly sliced fresh basil

Instructions

1. Position rack in upper third of oven; preheat broiler.

2. Heat oil in a large broiler-safe nonstick or cast-iron skillet over medium-high heat. Add onion and zucchini and cook, stirring frequently, until soft, 3 to 5 minutes.

3. Meanwhile, whisk eggs, salt and pepper in a bowl. Pour the eggs over the vegetables in the pan. Cook, lifting the edges to allow uncooked egg from the middle to flow underneath, until nearly set, about 2 minutes. Arrange mozzarella and sun-dried tomatoes on top and place the skillet under the broiler until the eggs are slightly browned, 1 1/2 to 2 minutes. Let stand for 3 minutes. Top with basil.

4. To release the frittata from the pan, run a spatula around the edge, then underneath, until you can slide or lift it out onto a cutting board or serving plate. Cut into 4 slices and serve.

Prep Time: 10 Minutes

Cook Time: 35 Minutes

Servings: 4

Ingredients

- 2 tablespoons extra-virgin olive oil, divided
- 1 small onion, sliced
- 2 cups small cauliflower florets
- ¼ cup water
- 5 cups chopped kale
- 3 cloves garlic, minced
- 1 teaspoon chopped fresh thyme
- ½ teaspoon salt, divided
- ½ teaspoon ground pepper, divided
- 8 large eggs
- ½ teaspoon smoked paprika
- ½ cup crumbled goat cheese or shredded Manchego cheese

Instructions

1. Position a rack in upper third of oven; preheat broiler to high.

2. Heat 1 tablespoon oil in a large cast-iron skillet over medium heat. Add onion and cook, stirring occasionally, until starting to brown, 2 to 4 minutes. Add cauliflower and water. Cover and cook until just tender, about 6 minutes. Add kale, garlic, thyme and 1/4 teaspoon each salt and pepper; cook, stirring often, until the kale is wilted, 2 to 3 minutes.

3. Whisk eggs, paprika and the remaining 1/4 teaspoon salt and pepper in a large bowl. Add the vegetables to the egg mixture; gently stir to combine. Wipe the pan clean; add the remaining 1 tablespoon oil and heat over medium heat. Pour in the egg mixture and top with cheese. Cover and cook until the edges are set and the bottom is brown, 4 to 5 minutes.

4. Transfer the pan to the oven and broil until the top of the frittata is just cooked, 2 to 3 minutes.

21. Baked Eggs with Roasted Vegetables

Prep Time: 25 Minutes

Cook Time: 9hrs 25 Minutes

Servings: 6

Ingredients

- 3 cups small broccoli florets (about 1 inch in size)
- 12 ounces yellow potatoes, such as Yukon Gold, cut into 1/2- to 3/4-inch pieces (about 2 cups)
- 1 large sweet potato, cut into 1/2- to 3/4-inch pieces (about 1 cup)
- 1 small red onion, cut into thin slices
- 2 tablespoons olive oil
- 6 eggs
- 2 ounces Manchego cheese, shredded (1/2 cup)
- ½ teaspoon cracked black pepper

Instructions

1. Preheat oven to 425 degrees Fahrenheit. Coat a 2-quart rectangular baking dish with nonstick cooking spray. In a large bowl combine broccoli, yellow potatoes, sweet potato, onion, olive oil and 1/4 teaspoon salt, tossing to coat vegetables.

2. Spread vegetable mixture evenly in the prepared pan. Roast for 10 minutes. Stir vegetables; roast about 5 minutes more or until vegetables are tender and starting to brown. Remove from oven. Spread vegetables evenly in baking dish; cool. Cover and chill in the refrigerator for 8 to 24 hours.

3. Let chilled vegetables stand at room temperature for 30 minutes. Meanwhile, preheat oven to 375 degrees Fahrenheit.

4. Bake vegetables, uncovered, for 5 minutes. Remove from oven; make six wells in the layer of vegetables. Break an egg into each well. Bake for 5 minutes more. Sprinkle with cheese. Bake for 5 to 10 minutes more or until eggs whites are set and yolks are starting to thicken. Sprinkle with pepper.

Prep Time: 25 Minutes

Cook Time: 1hrs 5 Minutes

Servings: 4

Ingredients

- 3 cloves garlic, divided
- 3 pounds ripe plum tomatoes, cut into 1/2-inch pieces
- 1 medium onion, finely chopped
- 4 tablespoons extra-virgin olive oil, divided
- 2 tablespoons chopped fresh parsley, plus more for garnish
- ¾ teaspoon salt, divided
- ½ teaspoon ground pepper, divided
- 2 large green chiles, such as Anaheim, finely chopped
- 1 teaspoon ground cumin
- ⅓ cup chopped fresh basil
- 4 large eggs
- ½ cup crumbled feta cheese
- Hot sauce for serving

Instructions

1. Preheat oven to 450°F.
2. Slice 2 garlic cloves. Toss with tomatoes, onion, 3 tablespoons oil, parsley and 1/4 teaspoon each salt and pepper in a large bowl. Spread evenly on a large rimmed baking sheet or in a shallow roasting pan. Roast until the tomatoes are shriveled and browned, about 45 minutes.
3. Chop the remaining garlic clove. Heat the remaining 1 tablespoon oil in a large skillet over medium heat. Add the garlic and chiles; cook, stirring, for 2 minutes. Add cumin and cook, stirring, for 30 seconds. Stir in the tomato mixture, the remaining 1/2 teaspoon salt and basil. Bring to a simmer and cook, stirring occasionally, until the tomatoes are mostly broken down, 6 to 8 minutes.
4. Make 4 deep indentations in the sauce with the back of a spoon and carefully crack an egg into each. Sprinkle the eggs with the remaining 1/4 teaspoon pepper. Cover and cook over medium-low until the whites are set, 6 to 8 minutes.
5. Remove from heat, sprinkle with feta and let stand, covered, for 2 minutes. (The eggs will continue to cook

a bit as they stand.) Garnish with parsley and serve with hot sauce, if desired.

Prep Time: 20 Minutes

Cook Time: 1hrs 10 Minutes

Servings: 8

Ingredients

- 5 cups shredded zucchini and/or summer squash (about 3 medium)
- 2 tablespoons butter
- 1 cup finely chopped onion
- Pinch of salt, plus 1/4 teaspoon, divided
- 1 ½ cups corn kernels, fresh or frozen (thawed)
- 1 ¼ cups no-salt-added cottage cheese
- 1 cup crumbled feta cheese
- ½ cup chopped red bell pepper
- ¼ cup chopped fresh dill
- 2 tablespoons all-purpose flour
- 1 teaspoon baking powder
- ¼ teaspoon ground pepper
- 10 large eggs, lightly beaten

Instructions

1. Preheat oven to 350 degrees F. Coat a 9-by-13-inch baking dish (or similar-size 3-quart baking dish) with cooking spray.
2. Place squash on a clean kitchen towel, gather up the edges and squeeze out excess moisture.
3. Heat butter in a large skillet over medium heat. Add onion and cook, stirring occasionally, until golden brown, 5 to 8 minutes. Add the squash and a pinch of salt; cook until very soft and dry; about 4 minutes more.
4. Transfer the squash mixture to a large bowl. Add corn, cottage cheese, feta, bell pepper, dill, flour, baking powder, pepper and the remaining 1/4 teaspoon salt and stir until well combined. Stir in eggs. Pour the mixture into the prepared baking dish.
5. Bake the casserole until the center is set and the edges are lightly browned, about 40 minutes. Let stand 10 minutes before serving.

Prep Time: 25 Minutes

Cook Time: 50 Minutes

Servings: 6

Ingredients

- Nonstick cooking spray
- 12 4-inch round thin slices lower sodium cooked ham
- 1 ¼ cups seeded and chopped roma tomatoes
- ½ cup thinly sliced green onions
- 1 tablespoon snipped fresh basil or 1 tsp. dried basil, crushed
- ¼ teaspoon black pepper
- ⅔ cup finely shredded Parmesan cheese
- 6 eggs, lightly beaten

Instructions

1. Preheat oven to 350 degrees F. Coat twelve 2 1/2-inch muffin cups with cooking spray.

2. Line prepared muffin cups with ham. Divide tomatoes, green onions, basil and pepper among cups. Top with cheese. Pour eggs over tomato mixture.

3. Bake 20 to 25 minutes or until puffed and a knife comes out clean. Cool in cups 5 minutes. Remove from cups. If desired, top with additional green onions and/or fresh basil. Serve warm.

Prep Time: 10 Minutes

Cook Time: 30 Minutes

Servings: 4

Ingredients

- 1 pound new or baby potatoes, scrubbed, halved if large
- 3 tablespoons extra-virgin olive oil, divided
- 1 bunch asparagus (about 1 pound), trimmed and cut in 1/2-inch pieces
- 4 ounces shiitake mushroom caps or other mushrooms, sliced
- 1 shallot, minced
- 1 clove garlic, minced
- 1 small onion, coarsely chopped
- ½ cup chopped jarred roasted red peppers, rinsed
- 1 tablespoon minced fresh sage
- ½ teaspoon salt
- ¼ teaspoon freshly ground pepper
- Fresh chives for garnish

Instructions

1. Place a steamer basket in a large saucepan, add 1 inch of water and bring to a boil. Put potatoes in the basket and steam until barely tender when pierced with a skewer, 12 to 15 minutes, and depending on size. When cool enough to handle, chop into 1/2-inch pieces.

2. Heat 1 tablespoon oil in a large (not nonstick) skillet over medium heat. Add asparagus, mushrooms, shallot and garlic and cook, stirring often, until beginning to brown, 5 to 7 minutes. Remove to a plate.

3. Add the remaining 2 tablespoons oil to the pan. Add onion and the potatoes and cook, stirring occasionally and scraping up the browned bits with a metal spatula, until the potatoes are browned, 4 to 8 minutes. Return the asparagus mixture to the pan along with roasted red pepper, sage, salt and pepper; cook, stirring, until heated through, about 1 minute more. Serve sprinkled with chives, if desired.

Prep Time: 25 Minutes

Cook Time: 25 Minutes

Servings: 4

Ingredients

- 2 tablespoons extra-virgin olive oil, divided
- 2 tablespoons diced shallot
- 2 cups rolled oats
- 4 cups water plus 1/2 cup, divided
- ½ teaspoon salt, divided
- ½ teaspoon ground pepper, divided
- 10 cups chopped collard greens (from 1-2 bunches)
- 2 teaspoons red-wine vinegar
- 1 cup shredded Cheddar cheese
- ¼ cup chipotle salsa, plus more for serving
- 4 large eggs, cooked as desired

Instructions

1. Heat 1 tablespoon oil in a large saucepan over medium heat. Add shallot and cook, stirring occasionally, until

softened, 1 to 2 minutes. Add oats and stir for 1 minute. Add 4 cups water and 1/4 teaspoon each salt and pepper. Bring to a boil, then reduce heat to a simmer. Cook, stirring often, until creamy, 10 to 12 minutes.

2. Meanwhile, heat the remaining 1 tablespoon oil in a large skillet over medium-high heat. Add collards along with the remaining 1/2 cup water and 1/4 teaspoon each salt and pepper. Cook, stirring occasionally, until tender, 5 to 7 minutes. Remove from heat and stir in vinegar.

3. Stir cheese and salsa into the oatmeal. Serve with the collards, eggs and more salsa, if desired.

Prep Time: 15Minutes

Cook Time: 15Minutes

Servings: 2

Ingredients

- 4 large eggs
- 2 tablespoons reduced-fat milk
- ¼ teaspoon ground pepper
- Pinch of salt
- 2 teaspoons grapeseed oil or avocado oil
- 2 tablespoons finely chopped shallot
- ½ cup boned and flaked smoked trout (1 1/2 ounces)
- 1 cup chopped spinach

Instructions

1. Whisk eggs, milk, and pepper and salt in a medium bowl until pale yellow throughout.
2. Heat oil in a medium nonstick skillet over medium heat. Add shallot and cook, stirring, until starting to brown, 1 to 2 minutes. Add the egg mixture and reduce

heat to medium-low. Cook, undisturbed, until the edges start to set, about 30 seconds. Sprinkle trout over the eggs. Using a rubber spatula, gently push and fold the eggs until fluffy and barely set, 2 to 4 minutes. Stir in spinach. Remove from heat, cover and let stand until the spinach is just wilted, 1 to 2 minutes.

Prep Time: 20 Minutes

Cook Time: 2hrs 20 Minutes

Servings: 6

Ingredients

- 16 ounces precooked shredded potatoes or frozen hash browns (thawed)
- 1 3/4 cups liquid egg substitute, such as Egg Beaters, or 8 eggs, beaten, divided
- 2 tablespoons all-purpose flour
- 1 tablespoon canola oil or extra-virgin olive oil
- ¼ teaspoon salt
- 2 cups finely chopped broccoli florets
- 1 cup shredded extra-sharp Cheddar cheese
- ¾ cup finely diced smoked ham
- ¾ cup reduced-fat sour cream
- ¼ cup minced fresh chives
- ⅛ teaspoon freshly ground pepper

Instructions

1. Preheat oven to 375 degrees F. Generously coat a 9-inch springform pan with cooking spray. Line a rimmed baking sheet with foil.

2. If using hash browns, squeeze any excess moisture from the thawed potatoes. Toss shredded potatoes (or hash browns) with 1/4 cup egg substitute, flour, oil and salt in a medium bowl. Pat the mixture into the bottom and 2 inches up the sides of the prepared springform pan. Bake until the potatoes are beginning to brown at the edges, 35 to 40 minutes.

3. Fill the crust with broccoli, cheese and ham. Whisk the remaining 1 1/2 cups egg substitute, sour cream, chives and pepper in a medium bowl. Place the pan on the prepared baking sheet and pour the egg mixture over the filling.

4. Bake the quiche until the center is just set, 50 minutes to 1 hour. Let cool for 15 minutes. Run a knife around the edges to loosen the sides, remove the pan sides and cut the quiche into wedges.

Prep Time: 25Minutes

Cook Time: 35Minutes

Servings: 6

Ingredients

- 1 ½ cups white whole-wheat flour
- 2 teaspoons baking powder
- ¼ teaspoon baking soda
- ¼ teaspoon salt
- 1 large egg
- 1 ½ cups buttermilk
- 2 tablespoons canola oil
- 1 tablespoon sugar
- 1 teaspoon vanilla extract

Instructions

1. Whisk flour, baking powder, baking soda and salt in a large bowl. Whisk egg, buttermilk, oil, sugar and vanilla in a medium bowl. Make a well in the center of the dry ingredients, add the wet ingredients and whisk

just until combined. Resist overmixing--it will make the pancakes tough.

2. Let the batter sit, without stirring, for 10 to 15 minutes. As the batter rests, the baking powder forms bubbles that create fluffy pancakes and the gluten in the flour relaxes to make them more tender.

3. Coat a large nonstick skillet or griddle with cooking spray; heat over medium heat. Without stirring the batter, measure out pancakes using about 1/4 cup batter per pancake and pour into the pan (or onto the griddle). Cook until the edges are dry and you see bubbles on the surface, 2 to 4 minutes. Flip and cook until golden brown on the other side, 2 to 4 minutes more. Repeat with the remaining batter, coating the pan with cooking spray and reducing the heat as needed.

Prep Time: 25 Minutes

Cook Time: 1hr 20 Minutes

Servings: 4

Ingredients

- 4 medium firm, crisp apples (about 1 3/4 pounds), such as Braeburn or Honeycrisp
- 2 tablespoons extra-virgin olive oil
- 1 large shallot, finely chopped
- 1 large clove garlic, finely chopped
- 2 tablespoons brandy or apple cider
- 1 teaspoon dried rubbed sage
- 1 teaspoon poultry seasoning
- ½ teaspoon salt
- ½ teaspoon ground pepper
- 8 ounces 93%-lean ground turkey
- 8 ounces lean ground pork

Instructions

1. Preheat oven to 425 degrees F. Coat a 9-by-13-inch baking dish with cooking spray.

2. Cut apples in half through the stem. Cut a tiny slice off the uncut side so the halves lie flat, if necessary. Using a melon baller or spoon, discard the core and seeds, then remove most of the apple flesh, and leaving a 1/4- to 1/2-inch-thick shell Finely chop the flesh.

3. Heat oil, shallot and garlic in a large skillet over medium heat. Cook, stirring, until it starts to sizzle. Add the chopped apple and cook, stirring occasionally, until softened, about 5 minutes. Transfer to a large shallow bowl and stir in brandy (or cider), sage, poultry seasoning, salt and pepper. Let cool for 10 minutes.

4. Mix turkey and pork into the apple mixture. Stuff each apple half with about 1/3 cup of the mixture. Place the stuffed apples in the prepared baking dish.

5. Bake until an instant-read thermometer inserted in the filling reaches 165 degrees F, 35 to 40 minutes. Let cool for 5 minutes. Serve drizzled with any pan juices.